Vegetarian Keto Diet for beginners

The Complete guide with Vegan Keto Diet and Plant-Based Diet for Rapid Weight Loss, Enjoying the Health Benefits of Your Life

Lara Meal

Table of Contents

Introduction

Congratulations on buying *The Vegetarian Keto Diet* and thank you for doing so!

The following chapters will discuss everything that you need to know in order to get started with the vegetarian keto diet for yourself. You may have heard about the keto diet and the vegetarian diet, as well as how both of these are meant to be really great for your health and your weight loss goals. However, did you know that you can actually combine them into one in order to really improve your health and ensure that you are going to get the best of both worlds? This guidebook is going to be able to help you get started on this kind of diet plan to see the best results in the process.

This guidebook is going to start out with an introduction to the vegetarian keto diet and how it is going to be different than all of the other diet plans that are out there. We will then move on to some of the things that you are allowed to eat, as well as the ones that you need to avoid when you choose this diet plan. In addition to talking about the general food groups, we are going to look at how you can make sure that you get enough fats and enough proteins to make this diet plan really effective.

From there, we are going to take a look at some of the health benefits that come with this diet plan, how to plan your meals, other tips for preparing the best meals while you are on the vegetarian keto diet, and whether or not there are any side effects or complications that you need to watch out for when you decide to get going on this diet plan.

The end of this guidebook is going to focus on a few other things that you need to consider when you want to go on the vegetarian keto diet. We will look at the importance of adding in your own exercise plan to enhance the weight loss and health benefits of this already powerful diet plan, some of the tips and tricks that you need to follow to get the most out of this diet plan, and then some answers to a few of those questions that you are sure to be asking when you are considering this diet plan above all others.

When you are ready to finally lose weight, improve your health, and make sure that you are doing what is best for the environment all in one, then the vegetarian keto diet is the right choice for you! To help you learn more about the vegetarian keto diet, make sure to check out this guidebook to show you exactly how to get started.

There are plenty of books on this subject on the market—thanks again for choosing this one! Every effort was made to ensure it is full of as much useful information as possible. Please enjoy!

Chapter 1: What Is the Vegetarian Keto Diet?

There are a lot of different types of diet plans that you are able to work with when it is time to lose weight and get in the best health of your life. Many of them tend to contradict one another. There are some people that focus just on eating lots of vegetables and other produce. Some like to cut out the fats and just eat carbs, and others go the opposite direction and will cut out the carbs all the way (or near it). Then, there are fasts, juices, and everything in between. With all of the information out there about diet plans and what is the best option for you to go with, the information can seem a bit confusing to someone who is trying to lose weight but feels like they are failing.

One diet plan that is growing in popularity because of all its health benefits, as well as its effectiveness for better health and weight loss, is known as the vegetarian ketogenic diet. This is a different kind of diet, and it is one that may make you scratch your head a little bit. However, we are going to spend our time in this guidebook focusing on how to work with this diet plan and get the most results out of it today!

You have probably heard about the vegetarian diet in the past. This is a diet plan that has been regarded as one of the healthiest diet plans out there for humanity to follow, as long as you choose to follow it properly and don't take it as a license to eat as much junk food and sweets as you would like. There are a lot of studies out there that find how the vegetarian diet is going to help you to reduce how likely it is that you will deal with some common diseases like diabetes and heart disease—and vegetarians are known to have some of the best health compared to any other group.

With that said, the vegetarian diet is not going to always be the best choice for everyone. Some people need to work with other things in order to help them to get the health benefits that work for them. For example, the ketogenic diet is actually seen to be more effective when it comes to weight loss than the vegetarian diet. Plus, it is able to help improve your blood sugar levels and triglyceride levels and reduces your risks of diseases like epilepsy, obesity, type 2 diabetes, PCOS, and some types of cancer.

Although there are all of the benefits that come with the ketogenic diet, there are still some health conditions to worry about with this one, and some people are also worried about some of the environmental concerns that come with this. The biggest issue environmentally that you will deal with is the idea that this is considered a meat-containing diet.

Dairy and meat from an animal and raised conventionally in a controlled animal feeding operation are going to be inferior when it comes to nutrition, but it is believed that they are going to contribute to climate change—and it is possible that some of the meats that you eat, mostly the packaged ones like salami and hotdogs, could increase your risks of various health concerns. Hence, it is best if you are able to avoid them as much as possible.

At this point, we are at a crossroads. We know that there are health benefits with the ketogenic diet and the vegetarian diet. However, we also know that there are some issues with both of these diets that make them not the perfect choice. From there, the question comes about what we are allowed to eat that will improve our health and help us to have more energy and is still good for the environment and our bodies all at the same time. This will then introduce us to the vegetarian ketogenic diet.

Definition of the Vegetarian Keto Diet

The simplest definition of this diet plan is that it is going to be a diet that is free from fowl, fish, and meat flesh that is also going to restrict the number of carbs that you eat. When you are able to stick with a diet plan that is like this, you are then able to reap all of the benefits that come with the ketogenic diet (the low-carb diet) while still reducing your personal carbon footprint, decreasing the amount of animal abuse, and improving your own health in the process.

Now, you are allowed to eat some animal products like dairy and eggs, if you choose. These are animal products, but they are allowed on the vegetarian diet because their production is not going to cause as much impact on our environment as some of the other animal products, such as farmed salmon, turkey, ham, and more. It is possible to even take this a bit further if you want to and just source your dairy and eggs from local and pasture-raised cows and chickens. When you learn how to support these sustainable and healthy rearing practices for animals, you are investing in the most humane and healthy animal products that you can.

In order to help you to implement this kind of diet in the proper manner, there are a few rules that you need to follow to make it happen. These rules are going to include:

1. Limit how many carbs you are allowed to consume each day. You need to try and reduce your consumption of carbs to 35 grams or less each day.

2. Make sure that all animal flesh is taken out of your diet. This means that all animal meats, such as poultry, fish, and meat, are cut out of your diet plan.

3. Pick out a lot of healthy vegetables that are low-carb to get the nutrients that you need in the process.

4. Your goal is to get a minimum of 70 percent of the calories that you consume each day from fat.

5. Consume proteins that are plant-based, including high-fat dairy and eggs in order to help you get the protein that your body needs each day.

6. If it is needed, especially in the beginning, you are able to supplement in some of the nutrients that you may be missing from the foods you are used to eating. You may find that supplementing with nutrients like

zinc, iron, DHA, EPA, and vitamin D3 can be the best.

7. Use a calculator in order to figure out the right ratio of calories and macronutrients that are going to work for you.

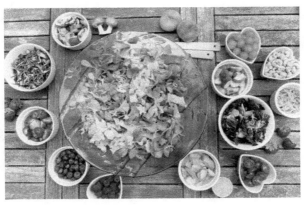

Limiting Your Carbs When You Are a Vegetarian

When you decide to go on this kind of diet, it may seem almost impossible that you are being asked to cut out how many carbs you are consuming. You are already cutting out your animal sources, which is a bit source of protein and fat for you—and now, you need also to cut out your carbs, and you need to be able to do this while eating plenty of healthy fruits and vegetables along the way as well. It may seem almost impossible for someone who is just starting out.

One of the biggest and most common mistakes that a lot of vegetarians are going to make when they go on this combined diet plan is that they are going to take on too many carbs. Primarily, this is because a lot of the foods that are favorites on this kind of diet plan are going to be high in carbs. Some of the higher carb culprits that you need to watch out for are going to include:

1. Grains. This means that you need to be able to cut out your cereal, rice, corn, and wheat.
2. Legumes: There are a lot of legumes that are usually allowed on the vegetarian diet, but they need to be avoided here. This means cut out the peas, black beans, and lentils as well.
3. Fruit: Next on the list is the fruit. You can have a bit on occasion, of course. However, you must make sure that you double check about the carb content and watch how many you consume because they are often high in carbs.
4. Tubers: This is going to be the yams and potatoes.

When you are following the ketogenic version of this diet, it means that you need to avoid all of the foods that are listed above. These foods are going to be so high in carbs that one serving is enough to take you from your carb limit and could take you out of the process of ketosis. This is basically the process your body will go into when you start the ketogenic diet, and it is the reason that you lose weight so quickly. Hence, staying in this process is going to be so important to ensure you actually get the results that you want.

At this time, when you look at the foods that you need to avoid in order to be a vegetarian, and then you combine it with the foods that you need to avoid in order to maintain ketosis and be on the ketogenic diet, it may seem like there is not much left over for you to enjoy. Before you start worrying that the only thing you will be able to eat when you do this kind of diet plan is lettuce and eggs, let's take a look at some of the food options that are available to you in this kind of diet plan:

1. Vegan-approved meats: This is going to include low-carb vegan meats that are high in protein, seitan, tofu, and tempeh.

2. Leafy greens: These are going to be low in carbs and can fill you up with lots of good nutrients along the way as well.

3. Vegetables that are found above ground: These are less likely to contain a lot of carbs, so they won't kick you out of ketosis in the process. Some of the options that you can consider include zucchini, cauliflower, and broccoli.

4. High-fat eggs and dairy: This would include options like eggs, butter, high-fat cream, and hard cheeses.

5. Nuts and seeds: Fill up on some of these as a tasty snack that will keep you healthy in the process. Some options that work here are going to include pumpkin seeds, sunflower seeds, almonds, and pistachios.

6. Avocados: These are a good source of healthy fats that are not going to kick you out of ketosis with their carb content.

7. Berries: If you need to satisfy a sweet tooth that you have, then working with berries is a great option. These still have some carbs, so don't go crazy. However, you will find that any berry—including raspberry, cherries,

blackberries, blueberries, and strawberries—can work well.

8. Sweeteners: You are able to add a bit of sweetener into the diet if you would like. Monk fruit, erythritol, and stevia are good options to go with on here.

9. Other fats: Fats are going to take up the majority of the calories that you decide to eat on this kind of diet plan. Making sure that you get a wide variety of them—ones that are low-carb, of course—can help you to see the results that you want. Going with avocado oil, MCT oil, olive oil, and coconut oil can be excellent choices.

How Do I Make Sure That I Get Enough Fat on This Diet Plan?

Your goal is to get about 70 percent of the calories that you need each day from the healthy fats that you are consuming. You want to make sure that you are getting lots of healthy fats, ones that are going to fill you up, burn your metabolism faster, and ensure that you are able to absorb all of the healthy nutrients that you are getting from other sources.

When you look at the list of foods that we have above, you should be able to see that there are quite a few different oils and fats that you can enjoy. Make sure to add these into your meals as much as possible. For example, cooking with some coconut oil can be a great way to start—or having some eggs for breakfast will give you the protein and the fats that you need to make it through the day.

If you are a bit worried about getting the nutrition that you need through this, then it is time to start watching your macronutrients. This is very important when it comes to following this kind of diet plan because it ensures that you are really going to get some of the results that you want. If you have too many carbs, or not enough fat and protein, then it is hard to stay in the process of ketosis and get the results that you want.

Figuring out your daily calories, or the goal of daily calories that you would like to stick with can be a great place to start. You then need to divide by the percentage of the macronutrient that you need. With the ketogenic diet, you want around 70 percent of your calories to come from fats each day, 20 to 25 percent from protein, and the last five percent from carbs. If you know your calorie counts for the day, then you will find that it is easier for you to come up with the macronutrient count in the process as well.

Working with the Process of Ketosis

We mentioned ketosis a bit before, but it is an important topic to understand when you are working on the ketogenic diet. The ketogenic diet is so effective—whether you combine it with the vegetarian diet or not—because it allows your body to get into the process of ketosis.

In the traditional American diet, we eat a lot of carbs. The body likes this because it is a fast source of fuel, but we are not really that effective at burning it all up. We waste through it like crazy, and then we want more. This is what brings all of those highs and lows in our moods and those cravings that we need to deal with. However, while the body is demanding more, we are not using up the supply that we have. Instead, it is getting stored on the stomach and around the body, causing us to gain weight and deal with a bunch of health problems.

Eating all of these carbs is not a good thing, and learning the best ways to reduce our carb intake and to ensure that we are able to still get the energy that we need, without all of the negatives and the endless cycle that is making us gain weight and get sick is so important—and that is where the ketogenic diet and ketosis can come into play.

The idea here is that the body, even though it really likes the carbs, does not need to have carbs in order to survive. It will do just well on fats to help us stay healthy. It may revolt a bit in the beginning, and we are going to feel worn out and tired in the process. However, soon, our bodies are going to adapt—we will not only lose a ton of weight in the process, but we are also going to come back with more energy than ever before.

The process of ketosis is basically when the body has finally let go of needing carbs for energy and relies solely on fats instead—but the body is lazy. If too many carbs are introduced into the body, it is going to revert back to using the carbs as a fuel source, regardless of how much fat we bring in—and that extra fat is going to be stored around the body as well.

Fat needs to be the primary source of food that we consume because that forces the body to rely just on that, rather than just waiting around until more carbs come in and feeling tired and lethargic in the process. Once you have switched over to the process of ketosis, it means that the body is running on all the healthy fats that you are consuming, along with your fat that has been stored in an unhealthy manner around the body.

The Negatives of This Diet Plan

For the most part, there are not any negative effects that come with this kind of diet plan.

You will be able to eat foods that are healthier and even lose weight while feeling amazing in the process—and if you have already been on the keto diet for some time and just want to add in the vegetarian option to help you get even more results, then the side effects are going to be even less.

There are some people who are going to experience a bit of something that is known as the keto flu. This is something that comes due to the keto part of this diet plan, and it is usually going to show up and sometimes be severe in those who have followed a really high-carb diet in the past and then tried to switch over to the keto diet suddenly.

This change is hard on the body. It is used to having that steady stream of carbs all of the time, and it is used to having it in high demand any time that it wanted—and then you turn around one day and take away that fuel source, causing it to panic, you to get irritable, your blood sugar levels to plummet, and you to just feel a bit crummy as though you have a cold or flu.

This is just going to last as long as it takes the body to start realizing that it can rely on your fat that is in the body and that you are consuming. Once the body starts to rely on that for its energy source rather than the carbs, you are going to see the flu, and your body and energy levels are going to start going back up.

Basically, when you get this kind of condition, it is just going to feel like you have the flu, sometimes with some more intense cravings that come with it. It is tough, but it is just the body reacting to the lack of carbs. It is not something dangerous that you need to worry about, it doesn't mean that the diet is unsafe to follow, and it is not going to last for a long time. Most people are just going to have it for a week, maybe two if they had a lot of carbs as a part of their normal diet.

If you are worried about this keto flu, mainly because your carb intake was high before you got started on the vegetarian keto diet, then taking it slow may be the answer that you are looking for. You can go through and just slowly limit your carbs. Maybe go from 200 grams a day to 150, and then to 100 and so on, until you get yourself to 20. This is easier on the body and will still get you some results along the way, even if they are not quite as fast.

As you can see, there are a lot of different options that you are able to pick when it comes to a diet plan, but none are going to be as healthy or as good for you as following the vegetarian keto diet. It is going to take some time to adjust to this diet plan and learn how to use it in the proper manner—but once you learn how to put it all together and what kinds of foods you are allowed to eat, you will find that it is one of the best diet plans out there for your needs.

Chapter 2: Which Foods Are Allowed on This Diet, and Which Ones to Avoid?

Foods That Are Allowed on the Vegetarian Keto Diet

The next thing that we need to take a look at when it is time to start on the vegetarian keto diet is what kinds of foods you are able to consume. You want to make sure that you are following the diet the right way and getting the health benefits that come from both—and since we are combining together two meal plans, paying close attention to the types of foods that you eat will make a big difference. Hence, let's take a look at some of the foods that are allowed on this vegetarian keto diet so that you can start to look and feel the best in no time.

Low-Carb Vegetables

The vegetarian diet is going to rely heavily on eating a lot of fresh produce to give you the nutrients that you need. However, you need to be careful about the types you are eating. Some of them—and too many of any of them—can put you above the allowed amount of carbs for the day. Knowing which ones are low-carb can help you out quite a bit because it will ensure that you are eating following the guidelines of this diet.

When you go on the vegetarian keto diet, make sure to try something new. There are a lot of different low-carb varieties of vegetables out there, and you can try to cook them in different manners. Working with butter or coconut oil to cook them, using lots of seasonings, and more can make a world of difference. Some of the best options for vegetables to choose that are low in carbs include:

1. Asparagus
2. Lettuce
3. Swiss chard
4. Collard greens
5. Kale
6. Spinach
7. Cauliflower
8. Green beans
9. Cucumber
10. Winter and summer squash
11. Broccoli
12. Bell peppers
13. White and red cabbage
14. Mushrooms
15. Garlic
16. Eggplants
17. Tomatoes

18. Onions

Fruits

When it comes to the fruits that you are able to consume on this diet plan, you have to be careful. While most fruits are considered pretty healthy, they are going to come higher in carbs than what is allowed on this diet plan. For the most part, you will want to stick with the berry family. These are lower in carbs but still full of the flavor that you want. Some awesome options that you can go with when it comes to fruits on the vegetarian keto diet include blueberries, raspberries, strawberries, and blackberries.

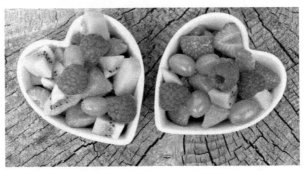

Condiments and Spices

As long as you read the label and make sure that you are not picking options that have extra carbs or sugars inside of them, you can go ahead and enjoy a lot of varieties of spices and condiments to help your meals taste better than ever before. If you are able to, try to make your condiments and spices at home, but if you read the label, you should be able to find some at the store that will suit your needs as well. Some of the options that you can make when it comes to condiments and spices that you can enjoy on this diet plan include:

1. Low-sugar or sugar-free, high-fat salad dressing
2. Sauerkraut without the sugars
3. Sugar-free ketchup
4. Mayo

5. Yellow mustard

6. Hot sauces

7. Worcestershire sauce

8. Coconut aminos and soy sauce

9. Pepper and salt

10. Lime and lemon juices

11. Nutmeg

12. Cinnamon

13. Cumin

14. Chili powder

15. Cayenne pepper

16. Cilantro

17. Thyme

18. Rosemary

19. Parsley

20. Oregano

21. Basil

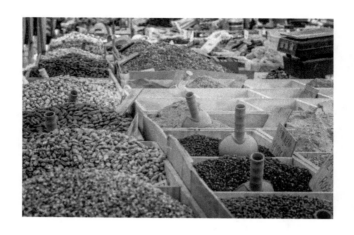

Protein

We are going to take a look at some of the protein sources that you are able to enjoy in more detail later on, but many people are actually surprised by the amount of protein that they are able to enjoy when they go on this kind of diet plan. There are a lot of great options that you are able to choose from when you go on this kind of diet plan. These are going to include:

1. Nuts and seeds
2. Miso
3. Natto
4. Tempeh
5. Dairy
6. Eggs

If you choose to go with any products that have soy in them, you need to try to stick with the ones that are fermented and non-GMO. If you find that you are eating a wide variety of these and your protein needs are not being met, using a protein powder made of organic rice or hemp could be the option that you are looking for. However, use it more as a supplement, such as adding to a nice shake for a snack, rather than as a meal replacement on a regular basis.

One thing to watch out for with this one is vegan and vegetarian meat substitutes. While these could be good when it comes to the protein and fats that you need, it is likely that they are a bit processed, and may contain too many carbs for this diet program. Always read the label and check to see what the carb content is for each serving. The best meat substitutes are not going to have any of the preservatives or other things that you need to worry about.

Dairy Products

It is a great idea to add in some dairy to your meal plans as well. Dairy has a lot of the good nutrients that your body needs, like calcium and vitamin D, along with healthy fats and lots of protein. Adding in a lot of options as snacks or sides to your meals can make a big difference in your overall health goals. Some of the options that you can choose when it is time to make sure you are getting enough dairy products are:

1. Mayo
2. Cottage cheese
3. Cream cheese
4. Heavy whipping cream
5. Hard cheeses, including cheddar, feta, Swiss, and parmesan. Make sure that you go with the full-fat versions
6. Soft cheeses like bleu cheese, mozzarella, Monterrey Jack, and brie
7. Butter that is grass fed
8. Greek or coconut yogurt

Fats

One thing that a lot of people worry about when they are first getting started on this kind of diet plan is how they are going to be able to take on so many fats. When we are used to hearing that fat is bad for us and that we need to avoid it at all costs, it is kind of scary to change that and try to eat 70 percent of our calories each day from these fats.

The trick here is to make sure that you are eating healthy fats. Do not run off to a fast food restaurant and say that it is all good because you are on the ketogenic diet. You need to fill the body with a whole bunch of healthy and wholesome fats to ensure you see the health benefits and the weight loss that you would like.

The good news is there are a lot of healthy fats out there for you to choose from. First off, are the oils. Some of the different oils that are great to mix into your meals, and even to cook and bake with, will include:

1. Avocado oil: This is a healthy monounsaturated fat. It is also going to come in with the highest smoke point compared to all of the other oils that you may want to use for cooking. This means that it is going to work so well when you want to deep fry, bake, and cook a lot of different meals on this diet plan.

2. Coconut oil: Next on the list is going to be the coconut oil. This one is a great option because it provides you with a bunch of fatty acids that can give you a lot of extra fuel. It is good for baking, cooking, desserts, and fat bombs, as long as the temperature is kept below 350 degrees.

3. MCT oil. If you have heard about bulletproof coffee, then you have probably heard about this kind of oil

because it is a big ingredient in there. This is derived from both palm oil and coconut oil—and it is going to be a special kind of fatty acid that is able to skip the normal digestion that fats go through and will head right to the liver to be turned into ketones for fuel. You can add this to your hot drinks, smoothies, fat bombs, sauces, and dressings to get the full benefit of working with these.

4. Olive oil: This is one of the best oils that you can use, whether in cooking, as a topping, or something else. In fact, there was a study done in 2018 that found how extra virgin olive oil is actually the healthiest and the safest oil to use in your meals.

5. Red palm oil: This is an oil that you probably have not heard a lot about,

but it is a great one if you need to add in some more nutrients to your diet plan. It is going to have a flavor that is like carrot, and a buttery texture, but it provides you with a lot of great vitamins and can be the supplement that you are looking for, while still providing you with the healthy fats that you need in the process.

These are just some of the oils that you are able to utilize in order to get some of the healthy fats that are needed in your diet. You can also choose from some healthy foods that have a lot of fats like dairy, eggs, seeds, nuts, avocados, and more. Make sure to add in some variety to your diet plan to help you get a lot of flavors and different options, and to ensure that this diet plan doesn't become too stale and boring to stick with.

When it comes to fats, there are other great options that you can choose to work with as well. You will find that olives, tempeh, tofu, nuts and seeds, healthy dairy products that are full in fats, and more can all be great options as well. With a bit of planning, and changing things up with some variety, you will find that it is easier than you think in order to get the fat that you need on this kind of diet plan.

At this point, you can let out a sigh of relief. You can see that there are a lot of different options when it comes to being on the vegetarian keto diet plan, and you will not be stuck just eating eggs and lettuce the whole time. There are a lot of options in foods that you can eat, and you are going to be surprised at how tasty and good your meals can be when you get the hang of it!

Foods to Avoid on the Vegetarian Keto Diet

Now that we have spent some time talking about the foods that you are allowed to eat on this kind of diet plan, it is time for us to take a look at the foods that you are going to need to avoid. With this kind of diet plan, the foods that you avoid are going to be just as important as the foods that you eat. For example, if you eat too many carbs, then you are going to get kicked out of the process of ketosis, and you will not be able to get the health benefits that are promised with the ketogenic portion of this diet.

Carbs

The first foods that you need to avoid when you start on this diet plan are the carbs. Carbs are going to kick your body out of ketosis and will make it hard to see the weight loss and health benefits that are promised with this diet plan. This means that all of your old favorites need to be avoided to get the health benefits that you need on this diet plan.

When it comes to the vegetarian keto diet, you need to avoid carbs as much as possible. Try to avoid pasta, pasta, bread, noodles, baked goods, and more. You need to stay out of the freezer section, the baked goods, ice cream, and more. This makes it easier for you to keep the carb content that you would need on the ketogenic diet as low as possible. For the most part, you should reserve your carb content on this diet plan for vegetables and fruits so you can get all of the great nutrients that your body needs. This means that you have to avoid all of some of your old favorites, but the results will be worth it.

Animal Flesh

Due to the vegetarian part of the diet plan, the next thing that you need to avoid is going to be the animal flesh. You need to avoid all kinds of animal flesh in order to stick with this. This means you should avoid ground beef, turkey, poultry, fish, ham, bacon, and more. There are other sources that you are able to choose when it comes to working with this diet plan, but you need to avoid the animal meats all the time.

Starchy Vegetables

There are some produce options that you need to avoid. For example, there are some starchy vegetables and a lot of fruits that will contain a ton of carbs that you need to be careful about. Things like sweet potatoes, yams, carrots, parsnips, peas, yucca, corn, cherry tomatoes, and more are going to contain a lot of carbs for their size, and it is best to avoid them if you don't want to worry about taking on too many carbs.

For fruits, the best options are going to be berries. These have the nutrients that you need, along with some antioxidants that your body needs to fight off diseases, without having to worry about as many carbs. However, you still need to limit these quite a bit if you want to stick with your carb content and to stay healthy. Most fruits are going to contain too many carbs so you will need to keep them to a minimum and only have them on rare occasions.

Sugary Foods

Any sweets, alcohol, baked goods, and more need to be avoided on this kind of diet plan.

The sugars are going to be the same as carbs to your body, and it is best if you are able to avoid them as much as possible. There just isn't much of a place for them, and you should avoid them when it is time to follow the vegetarian keto diet.

Sugary Beverages

One thing that we need to focus on here is what beverages you are going to be able to have when you are on this kind of diet plan. For the most part, you need to focus on is drinking lots of water, especially if you are new to the diet plan and you want to ensure that you are going to avoid some of the bad side effects that are going to come with it. Try to aim for eight to ten glasses of water each day to help you stay as healthy as possible during this time.

There are a few options when it comes to drinks, but you have to be careful about the carb content inside. For example, high-fat versions of dairy, such as milk, are going to be just fine with this one—but fruit juices, alcohols, and sodas are not. They are going to contain too many sugars and carbs in them that you will be kicked out of ketosis.

Sticking with green tea, water in all of its forms, and milk are the best options for you. If you would like to have a bit of alcohol on occasion, but keep it to one or two and go with options that are low in carbs so that you don't lose out on the process of ketosis that you are looking for.

Technically, diet soda is going to be allowed on this diet plan. The artificial sweeteners that are found on it are not believed to mess with your state of ketosis, and there are no carbs found in them. This means that you are allowed to have them on occasion. However, try to limit these and don't use it as an excuse to drink diet soda all day long. Your body really needs to get all of the hydration that it can from the water and green tea— and there are some studies that show that there could be some issues with drinking diet sodas on your health as well. However, having one as a treat on occasion is not going to kick you out of ketosis and can be good for you.

Alcoholic Beverages

The next question that you may have is about alcoholic beverages. You really need to watch these. While it is generally agreed that having some on occasion is not a horrible thing, there are a lot of carbs in these beverages and having them, even one in some cases, can kick you above your 20 grams of carbs a day all on its own.

There are a few different options that you can go with when you would like to enjoy some alcoholic beverages, but you need to pay attention to the nutrition label and plan your day around this—and no matter which option you choose to go with, remember that you are only going to be able to have one serving of these to stay within the guidelines of the vegetarian keto diet plan.

When it comes to the vegetarian keto diet, you have to make sure that you are careful with the foods that you eat. The foods that you eat and the ones that you avoid are going to be just as important as each other with this kind of diet plan. As you adjust to this diet a bit more, you will find that it is much easier for you to find the right recipes and meals that are going to help you to get the benefits of both of these diet plans and you will love the results that you are looking for.

Checking the Labels

One of the most important things that you need to do when you go on this kind of diet plan is to check the labels. You will be surprised at how many items and foods are advertised as being healthy or fitting into a certain diet plan that is just full of junk. Especially be careful of any meat substitutes like "vegan burgers" because these can often be full of too many carbs, along with issues with other bad stuff inside.

When you are looking at the label, the first thing that you should look at is the carbs. You want to make sure that the number of carbs in the product is not going to throw you out of the process of ketosis. A lot of foods that are promised to be healthy have a lot of extra carbs hidden in them, so check this out.

Once you know that the carb content is at a good amount, you should never have a single serving above 20 grams since this is your goal for the whole day and you most likely want to eat more than that for a day—it is then time to look at a few other things. Checking out how much fat and how much protein are in these items can help as well. Remember that you are looking to get about 70 percent of your calories from fat is critical with the keto diet portion of this diet plan, so check to see if that food is going to be able to help you out with that.

Next, go ahead and check what the sugar content is. Sugars and carbs are going to act pretty much the same in your body, and this is not a good thing when you want to stay in the state of ketosis. You want to stay away from things that have any added sugars in them. Some that have natural sugars, like berries and fruits, are fine, but stay away from foods that have a lot of added sugars in them.

Now go to the part that is below the nutritional label and see what they list out as some of the ingredients inside. Your goal with the vegetarian part of this diet plan is to eat foods that are wholesome and good for you. This means that you should not find a ton of preservatives or added stuff inside. If you see any of the hidden sugars, the preservatives, or any ingredient that you are not able to pronounce, then it is best to stay away from these foods and pick a different option.

When you are on this kind of diet plan, it is best if you stick with the outside rows of the grocery store. The closer you get to the middle aisles of the store, the more likely it is that you are dealing with foods that are full of all the bad stuff, the things that you do not need when you are on the vegetarian keto diet plan.

Instead, staying to the outside and going with the high-fat dairy products, the meat and protein substitutes (as long as they don't have too many preservatives and carbs in them), fresh produce, and more food that you need on this diet plan is going to be found in the outer aisles. In fact, you will probably do the best if you are able to pick out foods from the outside aisles and no more than a few in from there.

There are a lot of great benefits that you are going to be able to get when it comes to following the vegetarian keto diet plan. It takes some time to adjust to and get used to because there are so many parts, and it is true that you are going to need to cut out some of the foods that you are used to enjoying. However, once you get the ideas down and know how to make this work, you will find that there are a ton of great choices, ones that give you more energy, help you lose weight, and improve all the aspects of your health, without being as difficult as you thought in the beginning.

Chapter 3: Are There Any Health Benefits of This Diet Plan?

We have spent some time talking about the vegetarian keto diet and all of the things that you need to pay attention to in order to make this diet as successful as possible. One of the main questions that you may ask when it is time to decide if this diet plan is the best option for you or not is to figure out the health benefits that come with it. The neat thing here is that there are a ton of health benefits that come with following this kind of diet plan, as long as you are able to make it happen for you. Some of the health benefits that you will be able to enjoy with the vegetarian keto diet include:

Helps You to Lose Weight

When you follow this kind of diet plan, you are going to work to replace the majority of your carbs with fat to fuel yourself and your body. Carbs are going to be used by the body by being broken down into sugar. It is not efficient at burning through all of this, and it is going to be stored as fat in the body. However, when you go on a keto diet, you are going to replace those carbs with fat. The body is more efficient at burning through the fat, and you will be able to lose a lot of weight in the process.

As long as you are careful about how many calories you are taking in, and don't overeat, you will be able to burn through not only the fats that you are consuming but also the fats that are stored in the body. This gives you the energy that you need to feel good and can burn through enough to lose weight. A good way to speed up this process a bit is to make sure that your body maintains its ketosis.

Helps to Control Your Appetite

When you learn how to cut out some of the carbs that are in your diet plan, and you focus more on the healthy fats that you should consume instead, your food digestion process is going to be slow compared to when you were consuming sugars and starch. This is going to help you to feel full for longer and is a great way to eliminate cravings and control your appetite in between meals.

Now, you may notice that for the first few days of being on this kind of diet plan, the cravings do not go away. In fact, they may seem to intensify a bit because your body wants you to start eating those carbs again for easy fuel. However, if you are able to get through this time, you will find that ketosis has kicked in and the cravings are going to be all gone, while your appetite control goes up as well.

When it comes to reducing your cravings, especially when it comes to sugary snacks and other sweet foods that can affect your ketosis level in a negative manner, it is easier to follow a meal plan to help you not fall off your diet plan. It is hard to get through the first week or so, but once you are able to get through this time, you will find that following this kind of diet plan is going to be easier than ever before.

Can Improve Your Brain Activity

When you eat a lot of carbs in your diet, you will find that your levels of blood sugars will go up and down because these carbs are such an inconsistent type of energy. This inconsistency is going to make it really hard for your brain to stay focused, especially when you need to maintain that focus for a longer period of time. This is why we are going to feel tired and sluggish on a regular basis, even after we have just eaten a bit meal.

The good news is that when you switch over to a diet like the ketogenic diet, one that is going to focus on higher levels of fat, the ketones that are produced in the process are going to increase, and will provide the brain and the body with the energy that they need.

Unlike the carbs that you were consuming before, these ketones are going to be able to provide the brain with a consistent form of energy. This makes it a lot easier for you to keep your mind focused for a longer period of time—all day, in fact. The keto diet foods, along with the healthy vegetarian foods, are going to help you to reduce any of that cloudy mind feeling that you are dealing with, something that is more common with a diet high in carbs. It is also useful when you need to concentrate and can help to eliminate some of the symptoms of brain fog and mild levels of amnesia.

Provide You with Energy

It is true that the first week or so of being on any variation of the ketogenic diet is going to leave you feeling pretty worn out. You will go through a period that is known as the ketogenic flu. This is the time period where you are going to readjust to not having a steady supply of carbs to keep you going. You will be tired, have headaches, feel sick, and probably be cranky, all on top of a bunch of food cravings as well.

The reason that this happens is that you are going through a bit of withdrawal from the carbs. Your body is so used to having these as their main source of fuel that when you get rid of them, you end up with low energy. The body doesn't instantly look for the fat as fuel. It demands more carbs to help it out. It takes a week or so of not having the carbs before the body adjusts and learns that it is able to turn to eat fats to energize itself—and once this happens, you are definitely going to be able to notice a bit difference in the process.

But once that time is done, you will find that your energy levels are going to head through the roof. You will be able to get up in the morning and get things done, notice that workouts are easier, and eventually love that you are able to keep up with the kids and feel good, without wearing out and feeling tired by the end of the day. If you are someone who has been suffering from low energy levels, then it may be time to check out the vegetarian keto diet and see what a difference it can make for you.

A ketogenic diet, of any kind, is going to be able to provide you with a ton of energy reserves, much more than you need. When you are following a diet that is high in carbs, the body is only going to absorb a bit of the glycogen simply because it is not able to store it all as fuel. This means that you will need to continue to refuel the energy level to help yourself stay active from the start of the day to the end, even though you are eating plenty and may feel like you should not have to do this.

The good news is that when you start to consume more fats in your diet, just like with what you do on the vegetarian keto diet, you will all of the extra is going to be stored as fat—and since you need to have plenty of extra fat in order to keep your body going here, it means that you have plenty of energy, from the fat stores and from the food that you are eating all day long, in order to get through the daily activities that are required, and to help you perform any daily task that you need to get done.

Many people who are tired of not having enough energy to get through the day and who want to make sure that they are able to get more done will find that the ketogenic diet is a good way to get started. In fact, this diet plan is going to help you to get your energy levels up as high as possible through the day!

Helps to Lower Your Blood Pressure

Another benefit that you are going to be able to get when you choose to go on this kind of diet plan is that it can help you to reduce how high your blood pressure levels are. Blood pressure is a huge issue in the United

States. It is going to cause a lot of unneeded strain on your heart and arteries if you do not take care of it in the proper manner—and it can really cause a lot of other issues for your heart health as well.

Learning how to get your blood pressure down as much as possible is going to be a critical component to improving your health. The reason that you are able to lower your blood pressure with the help of the vegetarian keto diet is that you are limiting the number of carbs that you eat and increasing the fat content of your meals as well.

In fact, this is so effective that patients who have been diagnosed with high blood pressure found that their high levels decreased when they decided to switch over to the vegetarian keto diet. This has been so effective for some people that they were able to reduce or stop taking their blood pressure medications while they were on a diet, regardless of how high their numbers had been in the beginning.

Fills Your Body with Lots of Nutrients

When you start to eat the foods that are allowed on the vegetarian keto diet, you are going to fill your body with a ton of great nutrients. You are going to love how good you feel after adding these into the diet plan. With all of the healthy fats, the produce, and the good sources of protein, you are going to feel amazing in no time.

Adding those nutrients into your diet, even without all of the benefits of ketosis and the ketogenic diet, will do some wonders for your body. This is even truer when you get started on this diet from a traditional American diet as your foundation. It may take some time to get used to, but the detox that your body goes through when you are on this kind of diet can feel amazing and will help you to really enjoy some of the health benefits that we talked about before.

Reduce Your Blood Sugar Levels

Your blood sugar levels go through the roof because of the sugars and the carbs that you consume. Remember that carbs are going to be turned into a type of sugar when they enter the body. When you combine a lot of carbs with a lot of sugars through the day, you are going to raise that blood sugar up through the roof—and it is hard to fight this because all of those cravings start showing up, making it hard to avoid eating more and more of both the carbs and the sugars through the day, despite how bad we know they are for us.

When you start to cut out the carbs and only eat a few grams of them a day, you can help to lower the blood sugar levels. There are no longer blood sugars found (at least not in the amounts that they were in the past), and the cells can stop being as resistant to them as they were when the levels were so high. Because of this, the vegetarian keto diet is able to help reduce insulin resistance and type 1 and type 2 diabetes.

Helps You to Get Better Sleep

When you are able to improve a lot of the different health conditions that come with eating a poor diet plan, you will find that you are even able to sleep better. These negative health factors are going to really mess with how you are feeling, and the stress of how you are able to deal with them is going to really take its toll on you overall. When you can manage them better through a good exercise program and some healthy eating, you will find that your quality of sleep is going to improve as well.

With that said, you may need to adjust your sleeping schedule a bit to ensure you are getting enough. In addition to not eating the healthy foods that you should and getting a good exercise routine going, lack of sleep is also making it hard for you to get the health benefits that you are looking for. You need to make sure that you are aiming towards eight to nine hours of sleep a night to help your body recharge and to leave you feeling good and refreshed in the morning.

There are a number of things that you are able to do in order to help yourself get enough sleep on a regular basis. Setting up the right bedtime so that you get to sleep without all of the distractions do help. Setting up a good routine, turning off the electronics, turning the mind down, working with a dark room and some light music if you need it, and even keeping the temperature down a few degrees at night can make a difference. Your sleep is so important to your overall health and getting enough is only going to enhance some of the other benefits that you will see with this diet plan.

Gives You More Energy

One thing that you are going to notice when you decide to go on the vegetarian keto diet is that you will gain a ton of energy that you never had before. While it is true that your energy stores are going to head south for a few weeks or so while the body adjusts to not having a steady stream of carbs for fuel, once the body makes that adjustment, you are going to have more energy than you know what to do with.

As you can see, the vegetarian keto diet is one of the best things that you are able to do when it is time for you to lose weight and improve your whole health and life in the process. The above will be a few of the benefits and health perks that come with this diet plan, and you can easily see why so many people are in love with trying this option out.

Chapter 4: How Do I Make Sure I Get Enough Protein?

One concern that a lot of people have when they get started with the vegetarian keto diet is that they want to make sure that they get enough protein. Since you are cutting out a big source of protein—thanks to not consuming any meat or animal flesh—it is hard to get the protein, if you don't plan things out. The good news is that with a bit of creativity and research, you can easily get the amount of protein that you need in this kind of diet plan. There are a lot of sources of protein on the vegetarian keto diet, and some of the options that are available to you include:

Tofu

Tofu is a substance that is made out of soybeans and will contain a high amount of calcium and protein. The best part is that you are able to use it as a great substitute when it comes to meals that need fish, poultry, and meat. Although you may find that tofu often comes as mushy and soft, you are able to purchase different kinds, including kinds that are extra-firm. You should try to marinate it and season it before cooking so that it has time to add in those flavors and make your meals even better than before.

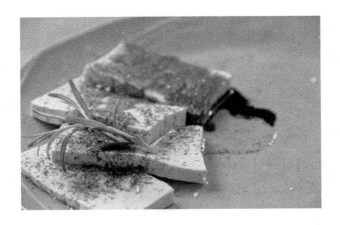

Tempeh

The next thing to consider when you want to make sure that you are getting plenty of protein into your meals is the idea of tempeh. This is going to be a fermented form of soy that has a firmer texture compared to tofu and is actually a bit grainier. This is a good option to replace any ground beef or fish recipes that you have. The only thing that you will need to do in order to get the tempeh prepared is to slice it, dice it, or even grind it up with the help of your food processor.

The one thing to remember here is that this product is made out of soy. For most people, this is not a bit issues, but some people have a sensitivity to it and need to avoid it. If you gain weight without an explanation, have dry skin, lots of constipation, are sensitive to cold, or have a lot of fatigue past the initial switch to the ketogenic diet, then it may be time to cut this food out of your diet and find something that can give you the protein that you need.

Seitan

This is another option that you may find useful when it comes to finding the protein that you need on this diet plan. Seitan or wheat meat is going to be a meat substitute that many vegetarians like to enjoy. It is going to be made out of seaweed, garlic, ginger, soy sauce or tamari, and wheat gluten. This is a type of vegan meat that has a lot of the different things in it that you need such as iron, low in fat, and high in protein.

If you are worried about gluten, then this product may not be the right option for you. In fact, the main source of protein that you are getting out of this is going to come from gluten. For most people, this is not going to be an issue because they are not sensitive to gluten—but if you do have this sensitivity, then seitan is not the best option for you.

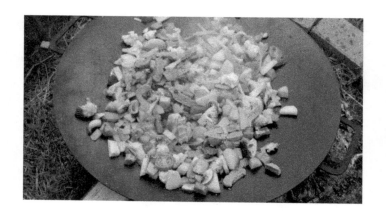

Other Vegan Choices

There are a few other types of vegan meat and even burgers out there that you are able to enjoy if you choose. However, if you want to go with these products, you are going to need to take some precautions and learn how to read all of the labels carefully. Just because something is vegan doesn't mean that it is healthy for you—and it is possible that some of these vegan and vegetarian products are going to be fine on these diet plans, but contain a lot of carbs in them so that would kick you out of the keto part of this.

If you are looking at the label and you notice it has a ton of carbs in it, or the ingredients look harmful, you see a lot of added sugar and carbs, or you are not able to pronounce a lot of the ingredients that are on the box, then do not buy this. There are a lot of good products for you out there that are going to have simple ingredients with a low amount of carbs, while also adding in the protein and your needed fat, you just need to be able to search around and find them.

Nuts and Seeds

Another place that you are able to look when it comes to helping you get enough protein into your diet is going to be the nuts and seeds. These are packed with protein, along with a lot of the healthy fats that your body needs as well. The nuts and the seeds that you should focus on because they are going to have the most protein in them for every 100 grams are going to include:

1. Flaxseeds: these are going to have 18 grams of protein
2. Sunflower seeds: These are going to have 19 grams.
3. Almonds: These are going to come in 21 grams.
4. Pistachios: These are going to have 21 grams
5. Pumpkin seeds: These are the best because they have 30 grams of protein.

However, when you are consuming these nuts and seeds, you need to be careful about some of them. They are going to be high in carb content, and you have to watch out for these when you are on the vegetarian keto diet, or you will get kicked out of the process of ketosis, and you won't be able to see the weight loss that you are looking for. Limit how many of these you have and keep your servings proportional, or you will be out of luck here too.

One thing to note when it comes to the nuts that you are consuming is the idea of peanuts. These are technically seen as a legume, but they are high in protein, considered vegetarian, and are low in carb content as well. You can include these on your diet on occasion, just make sure that you take into account the carb content and determine if you have enough carbs to handle this through that day.

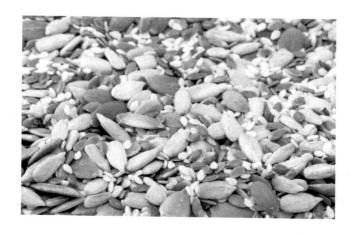

Protein Powders

When it comes to using protein powder, it is possible that this could give you the results that you want as well. You just need to make sure that you are picking out the right kind. When you go with one of these protein powders, you should go with grass-fed whey and organic pea protein isolate if you can because these are seen as the best option. These may not always have more nutritional value than others, but their impact on the environment is going to be less as well.

Adding protein powder to your day does not have to be difficult. You can make a low-carb smoothie for a snack or for one of your meals or add these to your meals in the sauces, to make some delicious fat bombs, and other options can really help you to add in more protein to your day can make a big difference.

Dairy and Egg Products

And of course, when it comes to working with the vegetarian keto diet, you also can enjoy high-fat dairy products and eggs. These are approved on the vegetarian diet and can provide you with a good source of protein and even healthy fats to help you meet your macronutrient content by the end of the day.

When picking out the eggs that you would like to consume, try to stick with free range options. These are going to be a bit better when it comes to the environment, which is a major concern for those who are going on a vegetarian style diet. In addition, if you are able to pick out milk and dairy options that come from animals who were pastured fed, this is better for the environment as well.

There are a lot of ways that you are able to add in more protein through dairy and egg products. Having an egg casserole, or just some plain eggs cooked the way that you like for breakfast can help. Adding in a cup of milk with your dinner or some Greek yogurt for a snack can work as well. These are surprisingly low in calories, while still providing you a good amount of protein that you need as well.

As you can see, there are a lot of choices on the vegetarian keto diet that will help you to get the protein that your body needs. Adding in as much variety to the diet plan as possible, and working to ensure that you choose options that are higher in protein and fat will help you to get all of the nutrition that you need with this diet plan, with none of the bad stuff along the way.

Chapter 5: Tips to Help You Prepare the Best Meals with the Vegetarian Keto Diet

Another thing that you may be worried about when it comes to the vegetarian keto diet is how you are going to be able to handle the meals that you need to make on this kind of plan. These meals may seem a bit complicated, and you may be scrambling around trying to figure out how you are going to get all of the meals prepped and ready to go in a timely manner.

This chapter is going to give you the help that you need to make this happen. You will see how meal planning and other steps will ensure that you are able to make healthy and delicious meals—without having to scramble around and try to get it all organized on your own. Some of the things that you are able to do in order to help you prepare the best meals with the vegetarian keto diet include:

Meal Plan

Meal planning is going to become your best friend when it is time to work with the vegetarian keto diet. This is going to make your life easier, will ensure that you have all of the nutrients that you need to see results, and makes sure that you have some tasty and delicious meals to eat on a regular basis.

Working with meal planning is going to be a bit different for everyone who decides to use it. You may decide to work with freezer meals or just prepping enough to make dinner easier. You may plan out one week in advance, or you can plan out a whole month and be really prepared. There really isn't a wrong way to do this as long as you pick meals you like and do as much of the work on them as you can ahead of time.

To start out with meal planning, you need to sit down and find the recipes that you would like to work with. Since you are working with a vegetarian keto diet, you need to pull out a few cookbooks that relate to this and then start to pick out the recipes that you would like to use. Write down the recipes and the ingredients that you need to use to go with each of them and start to make your own grocery list in the process.

When that grocery list is finished, it is time to head to the store. Take the list and try to stick with it. This is going to ensure that you are going to pick up ingredients that are healthy and approved on the vegetarian keto diet, and will help you to stick with what you need. It also helps you to save money because you just grab what you need, without having to grab anything else that can get costly.

Bring all of the items home. If you have time and the ambition, you can start on the meal prepping right away, or save it to do the next day. Your goal is to get as much done on this ahead of time as possible. This will ensure that you are able to keep things simple through the week. Make the casseroles, cut up the vegetables and fruits, and do anything else that you need.

Store the food items the way that they need to be stored. This helps to make it easier to pull things out as you need them through the week. This helps you to be able to have the healthy meals that you need—and it is as simple as that!

There are a lot of benefits that you are able to work with when you go on the vegetarian keto diet. Some of the benefits that you will love when it comes to meal planning, in general, and on this kind of diet plan, will include:

1. It can save you a lot of time. While it does take some time to find the recipes you need, go shopping, and get all of the meals together, meal planning is actually going to be able to save you a lot of time—and as you get better and more used to the meal planning and the recipes that you want to use, you

will find that it gets a lot faster over time.

2. It can help to save you money: Eating out can be expensive—and running to the store to grab something quick when you have no idea what to make for supper can cost a lot as well. When you plan your meal, you only pick up what you need. You can use discounts at the store and even purchase in bulk. This helps you to keep more money in your pocket while still getting to eat the good meals that you would like.

3. It is a lot healthier: Meal planning is going to help you stay healthy. You won't be eating out. You won't go to the freezer section at the store—and you won't throw together something because it is quick and easy without regards to how healthy it is for you.

With meal planning, you can look at your diet plan and make sure that everything that is needed so that you stay as healthy as possible.

4. It helps you to be prepared: You never know when there is going to be a night when you need to work late, a night when everyone gets sick, or when you just won't have time to get a meal on the table before you need to run off to another activity. Being prepared with at least a few meals ready ahead of time can reduce the stress that you feel during those times, helps you to get the meal on the table, and ensures that you will not have to waste time or ruin your health by going through the drive-thru.

5. It ensures that you will be able to stay on this diet plan: The vegetarian keto

diet is going to take some time to adjust to—and without meal planning, you may end up with some confusion when it comes to what to serve that night. If you plan your meal and have things organized, you will know for sure, because you already planned it all out that you are sticking with this diet plan and getting the benefits.

Doing some meal planning may take some time, and you need to come up with a schedule that works the best for you—but once you are able to put it all together, you will find that there are a ton of benefits, and it is going to become your favorite time of the week. The work is well worth all of the effort, and it helps you to get meals done and ready for those busy times in your life.

Check Your Macronutrients

When you are on the vegetarian keto diet, it is super important that you spend some time watching the macronutrients that you are taking in. Your goal is to make sure that you are getting enough fats and proteins into the diet plan, without consuming too many carbs and kicking your body out of the ketosis that you would like it to be in. This can be a challenge, but meal prepping and getting things organized ahead of time can make a big difference.

So, what are the macronutrient contents and the numbers that you need to stick with to ensure that you are getting the results on the ketogenic diet? First, we need to take a look at the fats that you consume. You need to take in somewhere between 70 and 75 percent of your calories from some source of healthy fats that you can find. This is quite a bit, and it is going to take you a bit of time to get used to, but you will love how good you feel, how tasty the meals are, and so much more in the process.

The rest of the calories that you consume need to be split up between the proteins and the carbs that you eat. The protein is the most important out of the two of these. You should take in somewhere between 20 and 25 percent of the calories that you consume each day from some healthy source of protein. This helps you to keep the muscles strong and can help you to fill up in the process as well. Of course, you should save the last five percent for the carbs. If you go too much above this, you are going to end up losing your ketosis.

To figure out how many calories these end up being, or how much of each one are you going to need to consume, you need to figure out how many calories you are able to consume each day. Once you have that number, you will be able to go through and calculate your macronutrients. Then use this information to help you figure out the right meals that are going to help you stay happy and healthy on this diet plan.

Freezer Meals

No matter what kind of diet plan you are on, freezer meals are going to become your best friend. You will find that these freezer meals are the perfect solution when you don't have the time to make a big home-cooked meal, or when you are just too tired to try and do it all for the night and want to have a break. You simply need to make the meal (or a few meals) ahead of time and add them to the freezer. When you are ready to enjoy them, you simply need to pull one out of the freezer and give it time to defrost before enjoying.

There are a lot of vegetarian keto diet recipes that you can make that will go well in the freezer—and you are able to make as many of these ahead of time as you would like. Some people like the idea of having a few of these on hand in case they get sick or tired, or when they need to throw something in quick because of a very busy night. Others like to make a whole month's worth of freezer meals to help them to save time and money and to make life easier since they already know the meals are diet approved.

No matter which way you plan to do things, freezer meals are going to make your life a whole lot easier. They are going to help you to have meals ready when you need it most, whether it is just one or two days a week or a whole month at a time. Since you are the one making them at home, you can verify the ingredients that are inside and ensure they are healthy and fit up to your dietary needs—and they can really help to make your life a little bit easier.

Find Your Favorite Recipes

Over time, you will find that you are going to start having a few recipes that are your new favorites. These are recipes that you need to hold onto. You will be able to reuse them from time to time, which makes the whole meal prepping adventure a little bit easier to work with. Instead of having to find brand new recipes each week, you can go through and reuse some of the recipes that you already have, and make those ones that you switch in and out all of the time.

Many people find that working with a meal prep schedule of switching meals around every month or six weeks, and then using a rotating schedule for them can make things easier. They already have the meals planned out with the recipes to go with them. They know which ingredients they will need and how much they are going to cost at the store—and they know how to make the recipes which can speed up prep time and cooking time in the process.

As you go through recipe books and work on your meal prepping, make sure to save any of the recipes you liked, or the ones that your family seemed to be particularly fond of. Then keep these around for when you need them. Pull them out on a regular basis or when you need to prep something simple and quick that you know the whole family is going to love.

Consider Sharing Meal Prep with a Friend

Doing a diet plan on your own is going to be hard to work on. You may feel like you are isolated and that you wish someone else was going through the same things that you were. Or maybe you just want to make the process of meal preparation a bit more fun, and you decide to choose a friend to do it with you. Instead of doing it all alone, have a day together in order to get some meals put together, share some recipes, talk, and just have a good time.

Learn How You Can Eat Out on This Diet Plan

The truth here is that it may be a bit difficult for you to find some places to eat out that are going to be vegetarian keto approved. While we have spent some time talking about all of the good foods that you are able to eat on this diet plan, most stores and restaurants are not going to have a lot of these options available. Restaurants like quick and easy, and it does take a bit of extra work to prepare for this diet plan. Plus, there are not that many people who follow a vegetarian keto diet, so it is not worth their time.

If you do go out, there are sure to be options if you take some time to look around and do some planning of curse. For example, consider going to a vegan or a vegetarian kind of restaurant to help you get started. They will at least cover the vegetarian part of it, and you can look through the menu before you leave to figure out whether you are going to be able to find foods that are also going to be approved for the ketogenic diet.

For the most part though, it is probably a lot safer, and healthier for you anyway, if you choose to avoid going out too much. Make some delicious foods and meals at home in order to get the results that you would like. You can always make some freezer meals ahead of time to help you out on some of those nights that are particularly busy and where you are not going to have time to finish your meal. Think of how much money and time you are going to be able to save in the   process!

Preparing good meals on the vegetarian keto diet doesn't have to be hard. When you first hear about this kind of diet plan, you may assume that your meal choices and ingredients are going to be pretty limited. However, as you explore with this diet a bit more, and learn more about what it all entails, you are going to find that it can provide you with some great tasting meals that are easy to make, and good for you, in no time. Use the tips above to help you to create the meal plan and the individual meals that you need to see success.

Chapter 6: Are There Any Complications with This Diet Plan?

Most of the negatives that you are going to experience when you go on this kind of diet plan are going to be related to the ketogenic diet part of this plan—and most of those symptoms are going to fall away after you get past the first few weeks with this diet plan. You will find that these can be irritating, but they are not too bad, and you are going to find them give up pretty quickly in the process. Some of the different complications and negative side effects that you may experience when you go on the vegetarian keto diet will include the following:

Frequent urination. The first complication that we are going to take a look at is the complications of frequent urination. Your body during this time is going to try and get rid of all that glucose that has been stored in the muscles and liver and doesn't need to be there any longer. There are really only a few ways to get this glucose out of the body, and urination is going to be the best. If you find that you are making more trips to the bathroom, it is not a cause for alarm. Just make sure that you replace all of the water that you lose.

Drowsiness and dizziness. During this time, you will find that there is a lot that the body is trying to release from the body to help you feel better. Some other things that your body will try to eliminate may include sodium, magnesium, and potassium—and when these head out of the body, you are going to feel tired and maybe a bit lightheaded in the process.

So, how are you going to combat this issue? No one wants to feel tired and dizzy all of the time, and the nutrients that you are losing here are going to be a much bigger deal. The good news is that there are ways that you are able to keep those nutrients around. A few of the options—such as eating poultry, fish, and meat—are not a good idea. However, you can make sure that you eat some avocados, dairy, broccoli, and leafy greens to your diet—and consider adding a bit of salt to your food to help with the sodium issue if needed.

The next issue that we need to take a look at is the issue of low blood sugar. If you are just getting started on a variation of the keto diet, especially if you were really into eating a diet full of carbs, then you may have to deal with low blood sugar levels. Your body has really become accustomed to having all of those carbs, and it runs into issues of knowing the right amount of insulin that is needed once you take away the carbs. It is going to take the body a bit of time to make the right adjustments for your insulin levels.

If you find that this is a really big issue and you are struggling with issues of blood sugar levels, then you may need to increase your carb content for a bit. You won't be able to get into ketosis as quickly, but it will help you not to deal with the issues with low blood sugar levels. Once your body has made the adjustments that you need, then you can cut down the carb content a bit more and enter into the state of ketosis.

Another problem that you can look out for is the cravings. There are a lot of cravings that can come up when you get started on any variation of the keto diet, including cravings for processed foods, carbs, and sugar. When you start any kind of diet plan that is going to focus on whole foods and cuts out all of the bad stuff, these cravings are going to be around for a bit of time. When you add in the fact that you need to eliminate carbs, and the cravings are going to magnify.

The trick here is just to make it through. This is easier said than done, but try not to give in to the cravings that you are dealing with. Have something there that will motivate you to do well, and remember the reasons why you are actually on this journey, and you will find that it is easier to get through all of those cravings that you are dealing with.

Some of the other complications that can arise when you get on this kind of diet plan, especially if you were following a high-carb diet beforehand, will include the following:

1. Constipation: This is a common issue that a lot of people will deal with when they go on a ketogenic diet. This can be helped if you choose to drink plenty of water to replace any that you are losing in the process. Any time that the body is not getting the water amount that it needs, it is not going to be able to function the way that it should, which leads to constipation happening. Also, include plenty of vegetables that are higher in fiber, and consume enough salt to keep this side effect to a minimum.

2. Muscle cramps: Just like with the fatigue and the dizziness that we talked about before, muscle cramps are going to be caused due to a loss of minerals. This means that you need to make sure that you are finding some keto approved sources to replace those minerals. Whether that is through taking some keto approved supplements or through your regular diet doesn't matter, as long as they are added in.

3. Symptoms of the flu: This is something that is known as the keto flu. You may find that during the first week or so of this kind of diet, you are going to feel irritable, have brain fog, trouble sleeping, being really tired, and having headaches. This is only going to last for a short amount of

time, and then your energy and your health will come back. The reason that you are going to feel this is because your body is going through a big change. Keep your body stocked with lots of fiber, minerals, and water to make the transition as smooth as possible.

4. Bad breath: Another side effect that you may end up dealing with when you are going on the vegetarian keto diet is bad breath. This is because of the creation of acetone, or the ketones that you have. It may be uncomfortable, but it is a good sign that your body is indeed going through ketosis. It usually only lasts for one to two weeks. So just make sure you keep around some breath mints to help you through this time.

5. Heart palpitations: Most users do not end having to deal with this problem, but it is still something that we need to discuss a bit. If you are someone who has lower blood pressure, then this side effect is more likely to happen with you. During the adjustment time, you may find that the heart needs to pump harder and faster due to the lack of water and salt that is in the body. So, of course, the best way for you to deal with these side effects is to salt your food and drink plenty of water.

As you can see here, the side effects that come with this diet plan are not life and death. Most of them are just going to be a little bit uncomfortable and can mean that you need to rest and relax a bit more when you go on this kind of diet plan. That is not necessarily a bad thing, but it is hard to rest all of the time in our modern world. But if you want to deal with them, then this is something that you need to prioritize for the first week or two of going on the vegetarian keto diet.

With that said, you may want to spend some time checking your salt and water intake. These are two of the most common reasons that you are going to end up dealing with the side effects above. If you are able to add a bit of extra salt to your meals, at least to one of them a day, and you can keep a large water bottle around to remind yourself to consume more on a regular basis, and you will find that it is easier to keep a lot of these side effects away so you can actually enjoy the health and weight loss benefits of this diet plan.

Chapter 7: Adding in an Exercise Plan

The next thing that we need to explore when it comes to following the vegetarian keto diet plan is how you can add in some good exercise to the plan to get more results. When it comes to weight loss and better health, the foods you eat (and the ones you avoid) are going to be very important to you. However, adding in that exercise plan is going to make a big difference in how well you are able to maintain the ketosis and keep your body in the best shape possible.

Exercise is good for everyone, and there are so many options out there. That means that you will be able to find a good workout plan whether you are young or old, in good health or not, or even if you have never exercised in the past or not. Don't let your experience or any other excuse be enough to keep you from starting a good exercise plan.

One thing to keep in mind, though, is that if you were on a really high-carb diet plan when you started this, the adjustment period is going to be rough. You do not want to go all in for that time because your body is already adjusting and not feeling its best. In fact, if you choose to avoid any exercise or too much physical activity during the first week or two of being on this variation of the ketogenic diet, that is probably the best.

It is recommended that you try to take it easy in the beginning. The vegetarian keto diet is asking you to make a lot of changes, and that is hard on the body—and since a lot of people feel kind of weak, tired, and sick during the first week or two of the diet plan, it is hard to imagine adding in an exercise plan. Take some time off work if you need, just do some leisurely strolls around the block to help you get fresh air, and take it easy as much as you need. You can always come in later on and add in an exercise program to your eating program when you are ready.

But let's assume that we are ready to get started with a workout. We have gone through the first few weeks of the ketogenic diet, and we are ready to add in the exercise plan to help us get our health even better and to see more results with the weight loss that we want to see. What are the steps that we need in order to make this happen?

When you are on the ketogenic diet, doing lots of hard cardio is usually not recommended. This kind of exercise is going to require a ton of carbs in order to be successful. Carbs can be converted into energy quickly and will help us to keep up with that intense activity for a longer period of time. Fat is a great source of fuel, but it takes a bit longer to burn up and convert into the fuel that we need to do some cardio.

This doesn't mean that we can't do any cardio. In fact, cardio is important to our health, and it is still encouraged when you are on this kind of diet plan. But you will probably not go out and run a marathon when you are on the vegetarian keto diet because you just don't have the energy and the fuel source that will make this happen for you.

There are some options that you are able to choose instead that will still give you the heart benefits of working with cardio, without having to worry about having enough carbs around for that kind of energy. HIIT is a great option to go with. This is high-intensity interval training, and it is going to include short bursts of intense activity with moderate paces along the way. There are different ways that you are going to be able to do this, but a good example is if you decided to walk around the block and then added some short 90 second sprints in there every once in a while.

These short sprints are going to be so great for you. They get the heart thumping and working hard. They take up a lot of energy. But since they don't last for a long time, your fats or the carbs that you were able to eat that day will be enough—and it is constantly asking your body to adjust all of the time between the fast and the slow.

HIIT can be so effective. In fact, it is often a preferred method of losing weight and getting fit. It is going to help you to burn more calories in a shorter amount of time. Depending on how well you do with this and the intensity level that you decide to throw in there, it is estimated that you are able to burn as many calories in 15 to 20 minutes of HIIT as you can with an hour of other kinds of cardio. Having more results with less time is always something that you want to work towards.

Of course, there are other options for working out that go well with the vegetarian keto diet. First on the list is the weight or strength training. This is the one that a lot of weight lifters and more are going to rely on, and many of them who really want to increase their strength and show some better results at the gym are going to start following the ketogenic diet.

Your burned fat for fuel is going to be perfect when it comes to weight lifting. It is going to ensure that you are able to help you to release the energy at the right time, and it will keep you from burning out too quickly. Whether you want to increase your strength or just slim down with some of the workouts that come with this, weight lifting is definitely something that works well with the vegetarian keto diet and should be done at least two times a week for the best results.

Doing various stretching exercises is another great option that you should consider. These are simple to work with and can be something you add in during those first few weeks on this kind of diet plan. They can open up your breathing, stretch you out, and just relax the mind and the body while reducing the amount of stress that you are dealing with in the process. This is what makes them so effective and great for you, no matter what stage of the vegetarian keto diet you are on.

Yoga, Pilates, meditation, and just stretching are all going to be great options here. The point is to give your body some self-love and a break, one that it may need after some of the more intense workouts that you do throughout the week. Try to spend at least one day, but preferably more, in order to help you to get the results that you want out of this.

Mixing together the three types of exercises is one of the best ways for you to feel amazing and get your health in the best shape possible. All of these can come together to improve your heart, help you to get better focus, releases the feel-good hormones that your body needs, and to lose weight while strengthening the muscles. Is it any wonder that a good workout plan is recommended when it comes to following this kind of diet?

Coming Up with Your Own Workout Schedule

The next thing that we need to focus on is the idea of creating your own workout schedule. Each person is going to come up with a schedule that is a little bit different, and the goal here is to come up with something that is going to work the best for your needs and what you like to do.

We talked a bit before about how mixing the exercises together and making some time for each one can be so important. Doing this is going to ensure that you are able to really work out all the parts of the body and will keep you in the best health possible. But, if you find that you can't get into a certain type of exercise or it doesn't seem to work the best for you, then that is not a good thing as well.

In order to start on a new workout program, as well as to help you get all of the health benefits that come with a good workout program, you have to enjoy it. The number one thing that you need to focus on here is finding a workout that you enjoy. Yes, you want to get results as well, but if you are not enjoying the workouts that you are doing, and they seem like a chore that you don't like to do, then you are going to get bored, frustrated, and give up.

Once you have found a workout program that you like, whether you stick with one that is premade or you just mix and match different workouts to fit your needs, it is time to move on to the next step. You need to focus here on finding the right time to work out. Morning, noon, night or somewhere in between is not that important. What is important is finding the time that works best for you. Pick a time that you are going to devote to working out at, and then stick with that no matter what.

And consider finding a friend you would like to work out with. Doing the workouts all on your own—whether they are at your home or at the gym—can be a little lonely. Why not turn this into a nice social event, one where you are able to catch up with a friend and see some great results in the process. You can both push each other to see better results. When one of you doesn't want to work out or needs a push to keep on going, you will find that having an accountability partner will make a world of difference.

Even with the good results that you are going to see when it comes to the vegetarian keto diet, you may also want to spend some time focusing on a good workout plan as well.

Working out is going to give you benefits that an eating plan all on its own is not going to be able to do for you. Make sure to think about which workouts you would like to go with, as well as when you would like to work out, and then go to work!

Chapter 8: Tips and Tricks to Get the Most Out of the Vegetarian Keto Diet

The next thing that we need to focus on when it comes to following the vegetarian keto diet is how to find some of the best tips and techniques that are going to make you as successful as possible. This is a tough diet plan to follow sometimes, and there are going to be more restrictions than you may be used to with some of the other diet plans out there. The good news is that the work is going to be so worth it in the long term, and there are a lot of tips that you are able to use in order to help you see the results that you would like. Some of the tips and tricks that are going to ensure you get the success that you would desire include:

Find Someone to Do the Work with You

Following the vegetarian keto diet is a hard one to work with. There are a lot of rules to follow, and that keto flu is going to be so tough on you that it is likely that you will think about stopping it altogether at least once during the process. However, if you can find the motivation that is needed and stick it out through that tough spot, you will find that it is going to be so worth it in the end.

One way that you can really work to make this process better and to help you get through even the tough times is to find a friend who will do the work with you. Maybe you and that friend can both agree to go on the vegetarian keto diet together, or maybe they are just doing the keto diet on its own. Either way, you both will experience some tough symptoms with the keto flu, and being together can make it easier.

When you have a friend who will go through the diet plan with you, you will find that it is easier. You can both support each other when things get tough, especially when you want to give in to some of those cravings in the beginning. You can both help each other eat healthily, avoid the temptations, work out, share recipes, and so much more. Things are always easier when you are able to do them with a friend, so why not invite a friend along and make the vegetarian keto diet a little bit easier.

Prepare the Snacks

During the keto flu, you are going to experience a lot of crazy cravings. Your body needs to have fuel to keep it going, and it wants you to rely mostly on the unhealthy carbs and sugars that you are trying to avoid right now. This is going to be hard when the body is adjusting, but one thing that can make it better is filling up on more fats.

This may seem strange, especially when the body is really craving all of those bad things. But your body will actually feel full and be able to fight off some of the cravings a bit better if you feed it fatter throughout the day. What this means is that before you go on the ketogenic diet, make sure to prepare a lot of snacks and extra things to eat that are going to be full of the good fats and the protein that you need. These will fill you up, provide the body with some of the fuel that it needs, even though it is fighting against you on this right now, and can help to chase a few of those cravings away to make the keto flu period a bit easier to handle.

Drink a Lot of Water

Water is going to become one of your best friends during this process. You will find that it is going to be the number one solution to a lot of the ailments that you deal with while on this kind of diet plan. Do you feel constipated? Drink some more water. Do you feel a headache or like there is some brain fog? Drink some more water. Are you not able to digest things as well, or are worried about how many nutrients are getting flushed out of your system? Drink some more water. Want to fight off some of the issues that come with the keto flu? Drink some more water.

There is not a single issue that comes with the vegetarian keto diet that can't be solved by taking in some more water. If you are worried that all of this water is going to start tasting bland, there are some options. You can add in some lime or lemon juice, you can work with bubbly water, and even some green tea can work for your needs as well. Just make sure to drink up as much as possible, especially during the first few weeks of this new diet plan.

Find Your Motivation for Getting Started

Each of us has a different motivation for why we want to go on a new diet and eating plan. For many people, it is about losing weight. Maybe you aren't that fond of how you look in your clothes. Maybe you are tired of not having the energy to chase your kids or to walk up a few flights of stairs to get to work each day. Or maybe you are worried about the state of your health, and you know that losing a few pounds could make it a little bit better.

There are a lot of things that you can concentrate on when it comes to going on a diet plan, and some of them may have very little to your weight. Maybe you have noticed that your blood pressure is high or you have entered into the state of being pre-diabetic. Some people want to get on a variation of the keto diet because they have heard how it is able to help them to clear out the brain fog and concentrate more.

As you can see here, there are a lot of different reasons why you may want to consider the vegetarian keto diet—and this is a good thing. But what you need to concentrate on here is your reason why. Why is it so important for you to lose weight or improve your health? Your reason has to be unique and all your own. Do not try to follow and copy what someone else has said or done. Come up with something that is all your own.

This diet plan is going to be tough. There are going to be times when you want to quit because you are not enjoying it or you want to give in to that dessert or carbs or other foods that you want to have. But this motivation, this "why," is going to help you to stay on track and will ensure that you are able to see results over the long term. Without it, you are just floating around and never seeing any of the results that you want from this.

Take It Easy While Dealing with the Keto Flu

Even though this diet plan is slightly different than just the traditional keto diet, it is still going to come with a few of the same side effects—and the worst one is going to be the keto flu. We have discussed this one a bit in this guidebook so far, but having a good understanding of how it works and how it is going to affect you can be important.

Basically, you are going to feel like you have the flu, with a lot of cravings for sugars and carbs on top of it all. This may not sound all that pleasant, and it really isn't, but it doesn't last that long—and if you are able to get through it, there is a good chance that your body has entered into the state of ketosis and you will start burning calories and fat like crazy.

During this time, the cravings are going to be strong. Your body wants those carbs, and it wants them now. You are going to want everything processed, comforting, carb loaded, and full of sugar that you can find—and on top of that, you are going to be tired, have a headache, be moody, and feel sick. It is not the best time in your life, but you can rest easy knowing that it is going to last for just a short amount of time.

When you deal with this flu, take it easy. It is tempting to try and keep up with everything that has to be done all of the time. But this is definitely a time period where you need to take care of yourself, and you need to try and not run as hard as before. If you are able to, consider taking some time off of work so that you can nap, rest, and just not move much. Enjoy some of your favorite shows, sit in a warm bath, and find ways to nap a bit more so that your body can get the rest and the relaxation that it needs the most.

Definitely, do not start this kind of diet plan when you have a lot of stress and big projects to do at work. You are going to feel miserable, and you likely won't get them done the way that you want. Don't plan a big trip or a lot of extra work at this time because you won't feel up to it—and do not start an exercise program during this time. Sure, exercising is so good for the body and is going to help you improve in so many different ways. But your body needs rest now, and you can get to the workout program later on when the body has time to recharge and get used to eating the fat for fuel rather than the carbs.

Get Ready to Plan Things Out

The vegetarian ketogenic diet is going to be almost impossible to stick with if you don't have a plan, and you don't take the time to meal plan ahead of time. There are just too many things to keep track of along the way. You have to worry about what you are going to eat, how many macronutrients that you need to have and in what amounts, how to cover the micronutrients, and so much more.

Sure, you can try just to plan it at the last minute. You could go to the store and grab a few ingredients and then hope that you will be able to pull out some great recipes to throw it all together at the last minute. You can hope that on those busy nights, or those nights that you are too tired, that you can whip something up fast or that you can find a restaurant that has foods that you can eat—

and you can hope that you are able to think through your macronutrients and remember where you are and how many to have and how to bring that all together.

If the thought of the last paragraph made you laugh or made your head spin, then you know that none of that is actually going to happen. Meal planning is going to be your best friend here—you just need to figure out the way that you are going to make it happen.

Meal planning has a number of benefits. Sure it takes some dedication, and you need to stay on track and make yourself sit down and do it. But it is going to make your life so much easier. You will be able to go through and pick out the meals you want to make ahead of time (while checking that it all stays within your macronutrient allotment to stay in the state of ketosis), You can then write out the grocery list that you need, go shopping, prepare as much of the meals ahead of time as you would like (in some cases creating the whole meal ahead of time and putting it into the freezer), and more.

When all of this comes together, and you are able to work on meal planning in the proper manner, you will find that it is going to make your life easier. There will be no more guessing whether or not you have the right ingredients all of the time, or worrying about the nutrients that you are taking in—no more panicking on those busy nights when you just don't have the time to make a complete meal, and no more worrying about whether you are staying healthy. Meal planning can get all of that done for you and more in no time at all.

Find Some Good Recipe Books

One of the hardest things to do when you get started on the vegetarian keto diet is finding the meals that you are going to eat. Figuring out the different options that you are allowed to eat, and that are going to taste good, when you are on this kind of diet plan can seem almost impossible—and when you see the list of foods that you have to eliminate to be on this diet plan, your mind may skip down to just two or three ideas, and you start to panic.

The thing is we tend to focus on what we are not supposed to have. When we see the list of foods that we need to avoid, we automatically focus on that, rather than focusing at all on the foods that we can eat—and despite the restrictions that come with this diet plan, there are still a lot of great recipes that you are able to make and that taste good.

This is where some good old fashioned cookbooks are going to come into play. You can also search online. The point here is to look through as many of these as you can so that you are then able to see all of the different options that are really available for you to enjoy—and there are quite a few. While you are meal planning, focus on this a bit and see what recipes you are going to like and enjoy the most on this diet plan. There are often some really great recipes that will work, as well as some substitutions that you can use as well, ensuring that you are going to see the keto results that you want, all while remaining on the vegetarian diet as well.

Restrict Your Carbs

The number one thing that we are trying to do when we go on the vegetarian keto diet is learning how to restrict your carbs so we can enter into the process of ketosis. In order to get into this state, and to stay there, you need to be able to limit your intake of carbs to 20 grams a day or less. This is not that much, and it is going to take some time to adjust, so a bit of preparation is going to go a long way with it all.

While some people are able to consume a few more carbohydrates than others and still remain in ketosis, starting with the 20 grams a day is the best option to see how things go, and it pretty much ensures that you will enter into this state. What this means though is that you are going to need to avoid a lot of your favorite carbs, including some that contain protein in them, like legumes, buckwheat, and quinoa. These foods, while high in protein, are also going to be too high in carbs to make this work. You should also be careful about the dairy products (check the carbs in them), starchy vegetables, and most fruits outside of an occasional berry.

Include Some Good Proteins

Protein is very important when it comes to your health, much less with this diet plan. It is going to contain all of the essential amino acids, in the right amounts, to help us sustain our lives. Combining some of the keto friendly low-carb plant proteins like eggs, dairy, seeds, and nuts can help to improve the amount of protein and the quality that you get on this kind of diet.

For the most part, you are going to need somewhere between 60 to 100 grams of protein when you are on this diet. It all depends on your age, your activity level, your body composition, and your weight. Most people find that they feel the best when they eat between 1.2 and 1.7 grams of protein per kg of body weight. The top three proteins that you can enjoy when you are on this kind of diet plan to ensure that you get the high-quality protein that your body requires includes:

1. Eggs: This is going to contain a protein source that is easy to digest and high

quality. There is also a good amount of choline, which can help your brain to function better. Just by having two large eggs, you will get 14 grams of protein and one gram of carb.

2. Greek yogurt. Greek yogurt is going to be full of protein, along with the magnesium, potassium, calcium, and a lot of the probiotics that you need to keep your immunity and gut health up and running. You will find up to 20 grams of protein in six ounces of Greek yogurt and just 7 grams or less of carbs.

3. Hemp seeds: These are going to be high in protein, rich in soluble fiber, and they are a great source of omega-3 fatty acids, potassium, and magnesium. You will find that in an

ounce of hemp seeds, you will find one gram of carbs and 9 grams of protein.

Try to Get in One to Three Servings of Vegetables, But Keep Them Low-Carb

When you do eat carbs, try to get them from a lot of healthy vegetables. There are a lot of options that are going to be low in carbs, helping you to get a ton of nutrients in them without all of the guilt. There are a lot of vegetables that can be considered keto friendly. Plus, they give you a lot of fiber while filling the rest of your micronutrients as well.

Use Healthy Oils for Dressings and Cooking

Healthy oils can be one of the best and easiest ways for you to get in the fats that you need on the vegetarian keto diet. You will find that these healthy fats are going to taste great, will improve the texture of the food, and can ensure that you will stay full and happy for hours to come. Plus, when you pick out the right ones, they will ensure that your body is able to properly absorb all of those fat soluble vitamins that you really need, including Vitamins A, D, E, and K.

Fats are going to be the main source of your calories when you are on this kind of diet plan. This is why it is so important to choose the types that are the healthiest. Seed oils and vegetable oils are going to be ones that you need to avoid because they have been processed and are linked to inflammation throughout the body. This means that on the vegetarian keto diet, you need to avoid some options for oils like canola oil, corn oil, safflower oil, and sunflower oil.

Instead, you need to choose the healthy oils to help you out. Options like avocado oil, olive oil, coconut oil, ghee, and butter can be healthy fats and condiments for this diet plan. They are perfect as condiments and salad dressings, and they can even help with meal preparation when you are cooking.

Remember the Spices and Herbs

When you are on the vegetarian keto diet, remember that you can easily use a lot of spices and herbs in your diet plan. These help you to really get some more flavoring into the diet, while not adding in any of the carbs that you can find with some of the other condiments that you may try to use. Herbs and spices are going to help you to increase how much variety is found here while adding in a few more micronutrients to the body.

Of course, you need to try out some of the ones that are well-known because there are a ton of recipes that include them, like cinnamon, rosemary, and basil. But if you need to add in a bit more flavoring and fun to your meals, don't be scared to look outside of these and see which cool combinations you are able to find. You may be surprised to find out which herb or spice is going to become your new favorite.

Avoiding Any Nutrient Deficiencies

One thing that you need to focus on when it comes to this kind of diet plan is making sure that you get the nutrients that you are looking for. It is easy to fall prey to just eating one type of food all of the time, or not paying attention to what you are eating throughout the day. This may seem easier, but it is going to become boring after some time, and it is going to make you miss out on some of the great nutrients that your body needs so much.

When you are on a simple vegetarian diet plan, you are going to rely heavily on legume and grains in order to get a lot of the micronutrients that you need. When you restrict these foods, along with the seafood and meat sources that are needed on the vegetarian diet, it is going to make it hard to get some of the nutrients that you need.

Now, there are plenty of foods out there that can provide you with these nutrients, but you have to be proactive about making sure that you get them there. When you take the time to manage your micronutrient intake with good quality vegetarian protein sources, and plenty of low-carb vegetables, you will be able to keep this in line.

In the beginning, you may want to consider adding in a supplement to help you get some of the nutrients that you really need. There is a challenge to learn how to get these all in, and you don't want to have your body suffering in the process either. Making sure that you get some important nutrients, like magnesium, potassium, zinc, vitamin D, vitamin B12, calcium, iron, and omega-3 fatty acids, will make things a lot easier in the long run.

Following the vegetarian keto diet is one that takes some time and patience in order to see the results that you would like. It is not going to come naturally, and you really need to learn how to think through the foods that you are eating and the meals that you plan to create. You may find that it is hard to get started, but over time, you will be so glad that you did. Follow the tips that are above, and you will see the results in no time while feeling amazing about your health all at the same time!

Chapter 9: Q & A About the Vegetarian Keto Diet

Now that we have spent a bit of time talking about the vegetarian keto diet a bit and know more about how it is going to provide you with all of the health benefits that you need, it is time to look at a few of the questions that you are likely to ask when you decide to go on this kind of diet.

It is normal to have questions. This is a diet plan that a lot of people may not think about ahead of time, and it is quite a bit different than a lot of the other ones that you may have tried in the past. This is probably a good thing because it ensures that you will really lose the weight that you would like. Some of the questions that you may have when it comes to starting the vegetarian keto diet include:

Why Should I Consider Going on the Vegetarian Keto Diet Plan?

There are a lot of different reasons why you will want to consider going on this kind of diet plan. Sure, there are a lot of different diet plans that are available and can make a lot of promises, but none are going to be as effective as the vegetarian keto diet that we have been talking about in this guidebook. Some of the great health benefits that you are going to be able to enjoy when you go on this kind of diet plan includes:

1. Losing weight: This is the number one reason why people will choose to go on the vegetarian keto diet. They like that

they are switching over to foods that are whole and good for them. They like that the foods are going to give them all of the nutrients that they need— and they like that this all comes together, along with reduced calorie counts, in order to help you to lose weight.

2. Improve your blood pressure: Thanks to the fact that you are focusing on fewer sugars and carbs (which are more likely to cause issues with the heart than fats) and that you focus on healthy fats, you will be able to improve your blood pressure. Think about how great this is going to be for your whole heart when you can do this.

3. Reduces your blood sugar levels: Since you are reducing the number of

sugars, and the number of carbs, which are converted into sugars in the body, you are naturally going to reduce the amount of blood sugar levels that you are dealing with.

4. A better amount of focus: When you clear out the carbs that you are working with, and when you no longer have to deal with the sugar highs and lows, the better you are able to focus.

5. Help out the environment: When you add in the vegetarian part of the diet plan to the mix, not only are you getting all of the health benefits that come with the keto diet, you are also going to get a ton of benefits like helping the environment through the vegetarian diet. You will help reduce your carbon footprint, and you stop supporting animal mills and all of the

bad stuff that happens from raising animals.

As you can see, there are a lot of benefits that come with the vegetarian keto diet. It is one of the best diet plans that you can choose to work with because of its great tasting foods that are going to appeal to everyone!

Why Is Ketosis So Important?

We have spent some time in this guidebook talking about the process of ketosis. It is a very important part of starting the ketogenic diet. If you are never able to get into the process of ketosis, you are going to never really see the weight loss, and other health benefits, that you want with this diet plan—and this is a tough diet plan to follow. You don't want to put in all of that work and never get the results that you are looking for in the process.

First, we need to take a look at what the process of ketosis is all about. This is basically when your body is going to change from relying on carbs for fuel and switch over to relying on your fats—both those in your body and those being consumed in your diet—in order to help you to have energy and make it through the day.

This process is going to take a bit of time to accomplish. It isn't instant, especially since the body likes to be able to rely on the carbs and is going to fight with this one a bit—but if you follow the allowed and not allowed foods that we talked about earlier as strictly as possible, then you will enter into ketosis after a few weeks, and you will start to feel so much better in the long run.

There are a few different methods that you can use in order to check out how the process of ketosis is going. You can get a few testing tools that are going to help you to really see if you are in ketosis. Some are going to use your spit, and others may use urine to help you tell. You should use these in the first few weeks of the diet plan to make sure that you are entering into that process—and then you need to do it on occasion in order to make sure that you are staying in that process over time.

Now, if you are on this diet plan and you find that your results are not as prevalent as you had thought they should be or they seem to stall. The biggest reason that you may not be seeing the results is that you are not in ketosis—and often, that is because your carb intake is higher than it should be.

It may be time to relook at how many carbs you are taking in each day, and determining if the number is too high. Be honest with yourself here. You may have lost track of your macronutrient counts, and find that you are just estimating the counts and that you are taking in too many carbs. If this is the case, then it is time to get back to counting the nutrients again, and cutting down the carbs again.

The process of ketosis is going to be one of your main goals when you are working with the vegetarian keto diet plan. Without this, you are doing a lot of potential work without actually seeing any of the results that you really want. Once you enter into this kind of process, you will find that your metabolism speeds up, your cravings go away, and your energy levels go up while you lose weight at the same time.

Is This Diet Plan Too Hard to Get Started On?

One thing that a lot of people are worried about when they are looking to get started on the vegetarian keto diet plan is whether it is going to be too hard to follow. They see the fact that this is a combined diet plan, one that has two different diets that you have to follow. This means two different meal plans, two different sets of rules, and so much more. Just the thought can make a lot of people nervous along the way as well.

This diet plan is going to take a little bit of work. But that is what makes it so successful to work with. You are not going to be able to just walk in with the idea that this is going to be easy and you can eat everything that you would like. This is what got you to your present health and has driven you to want to lose weight, in the first place. Having some rules and guidelines in place are going to make a big difference in how healthy you are going to be when you get started on this diet plan.

If the idea of a little challenge scares you from this diet plan, then it is time to change your perspective a little bit. You need to really think through whether you are really ready to lose weight, and improve all of the different aspects of your diet plan in order to help you to feel better. For some people, this is too much. But you have gotten this far in this guidebook. You are ready for a change—and you *can* do it!

Just take it one step at a time, and one day at a time as much as you can. There are going to be days when it seems really easy, and the results that you are seeing will propel you forward to work even more and stick with it—and then there are going to be days when things get more difficult, and you even fall off. That is perfectly normal with anything that we do in our lives. If you fall, just get back up, find your motivation, and just restart. Over time, you will get the results that you want, and you will see that the vegetarian keto diet has become a regular part of your life.

Does the Keto Diet Work Without Exercising?

You will find that the vegetarian keto diet is going to be really successful, even without exercising. Of course, before you try to see these results, you have to make sure that your daily calories are at a safe level that you will burn more than consume. The keto diet part of this isn't going to be any different than any of the other dieting methods in the idea that you have to create a deficit of calories in order to lose weight.

The ketogenic diet can be really successful on its own when it comes to helping you to lose a lot of weight. Plus, it is going to be wonderful at helping you to increase a lot of other aspects of your health over time. When you add it into some of the health consciousness that comes with the vegetarian diet as well, it is likely that you will be able to lose a lot of weight when you decide to go on this kind of diet plan.

With that said, if you really want to see some of the results, and you are interested in toning and looking better while also losing weight in the process, then you need to add in some form of exercise on a regular basis. There are a lot of different options that you can choose when it comes to a healthy and effective diet and exercise program, you just need to stick with it and find the right amount that works for your needs.

Am I Going to Miss Out on a Lot of the Nutrition That I Need?

The next thing that we need to take a look at is the idea of whether or not the ketogenic diet, or the vegetarian diet, will be bad for you, especially when you decide to combine the two of them together. Many people worry that when they are combining a diet plan that cuts out all animal products, with one that is going to cut out most of your carbs, you are going to end up missing out on a lot of the nutrition that you are looking to get for your body.

The truth is, you can get all of the nutrients that you need while on the vegetarian ketogenic diet, but you do need to go through and actually do some planning. You have to actually think through the meals that you are going to eat, make sure that you have a lot of variety in the meals, and really double check that your macronutrients are in place.

There are a lot of different groups of foods that you are going to be eliminating when you go on this diet plan. This is going to help improve your health and help you to lose a lot of weight. But you need to be careful and actually plan out the work that you are going to do with this one. There are lots of options that come with this diet plan that allows you to get a ton of healthy nutrients, but you are cutting out on many of the foods that you are used to. And this makes it very easy for you to run into trouble because you need to really think through your meals.

As we showed in this guidebook, there are a lot of ways to make sure you get your carbs, protein, and fats on this kind of diet plan. But you do need to plan it out. You aren't getting as much freedom in choices. This makes the work harder. But if you plan things out, learn how to count your nutrients, and pay attention to what you are eating, there is no reason that you aren't going to be able to get the health benefits that you are looking for with this kind of diet plan.

What Are Some of the Drinks That You Are Going to Be Allowed to Have?

The next question that we are going to need to discuss on this is what kinds of drinks, outside of the obvious water to help with some of the negative side effects that can come with the beginning of this diet plan, that you are allowed to have here.

The good news here is that there are going to be a few different types of beverages that you are able to have when you decide to go on the vegetarian keto diet plan. Some of the options, outside of water, can include tea, coffee, and even some kinds of alcoholic drinks (check the carb content on them before you start), can work on this kind of diet plan. Some of the alcohols that do well with this diet plan, as long as you double check how many carbs in them and make sure that you are not having too much of them, include beer that is low carb, red and white wine, and clear spirits.

There will be a lot of drinks that you need to avoid when you decide to go on the vegetarian keto diet plan. Things like most alcoholic beverages, energy drinks, sports drinks, sweet teas, sodas, and fruit juices need to be kicked out. These are not going to provide you with the health benefits that you are looking for, and are going to be too high in carbs and sugars that need to be avoided.

Next on the list is the idea of diet sodas. Many people wonder if they are allowed to have any diet sodas when they are on this kind of plan. Technically, when you are on the vegetarian keto diet plan, these artificially sweetened beverages are going to be approved. They aren't going to have any calories or carbs, and this means that you are able to fit them into the diet.

However, just because they technically fit in with the keto status that you are looking at, it is probably not the smartest idea to make them a regular part of your diet. Having one on occasion is going to be just fine. But having them all of the time can make things more difficult. The compounds that are found in a lot of these diet sodas are going to compromise the health of your gut, and you should just have them as a way to satisfy some of the cravings that you have on occasion, rather than having them all of the time.

And finally, we need to take a look at your caffeine intake. We have already talked about diet sodas and coffees, so it probably makes sense that you are allowed to have some caffeine on occasion. Since this is not a carbohydrate, it is fine to have it on this kind of diet plan. Caffeine pills (although these should be taken sparingly if at all), coffee with some milk, and black coffee are just fine when you are on this diet plan. Just remember to not add in any sugar to the coffee in the morning, and you are just fine.

As you can see, there are a lot of things to learn when it is time to get started on the vegetarian keto diet. It is a great way for you to lose a lot of weight, improve your memory, work on your heart health, and just improve so many different aspects when it comes to all the parts of your health. Following some of these suggestions an ensure that you are going to see more of the results that you are looking for with this kind of diet plan.

Conclusion

Thank you for making it through to the end of *The Vegetarian Keto Diet*! Let's hope it was informative and able to provide you with all of the tools you need to achieve your goals—whatever they may be.

The next step is to start on this diet plan and see some of the great results that are going to come with it. There are a lot of benefits that come with this kind of diet plan, and it is definitely not as hard to accomplish as you may think in the beginning. This guidebook will show you exactly how you can eat and feel amazing when you go on this combination diet plan.

This guidebook took some time to discuss all of the things that you need to know when you want to get started on this kind of diet plan. There is just so much to love about it, and the simplicity that comes with it is going to be pretty amazing as well. We talked about all of the basics, how to make sure that you eat the right kinds of foods, and so much more.

Now that you know a bit more about the vegetarian keto diet and all of the health benefits, the environmental benefits, and more—make sure to follow the advice and tips in this guidebook to help you get the most out of this diet plan.

Finally, if you found this book useful in any way, a review on Amazon is always appreciated!

CPSIA information can be obtained
at www.ICGtesting.com
Printed in the USA
BVHW041519220221
600777BV00006B/460

9 781911 684237